krazy keto cookbook

for serious foodies

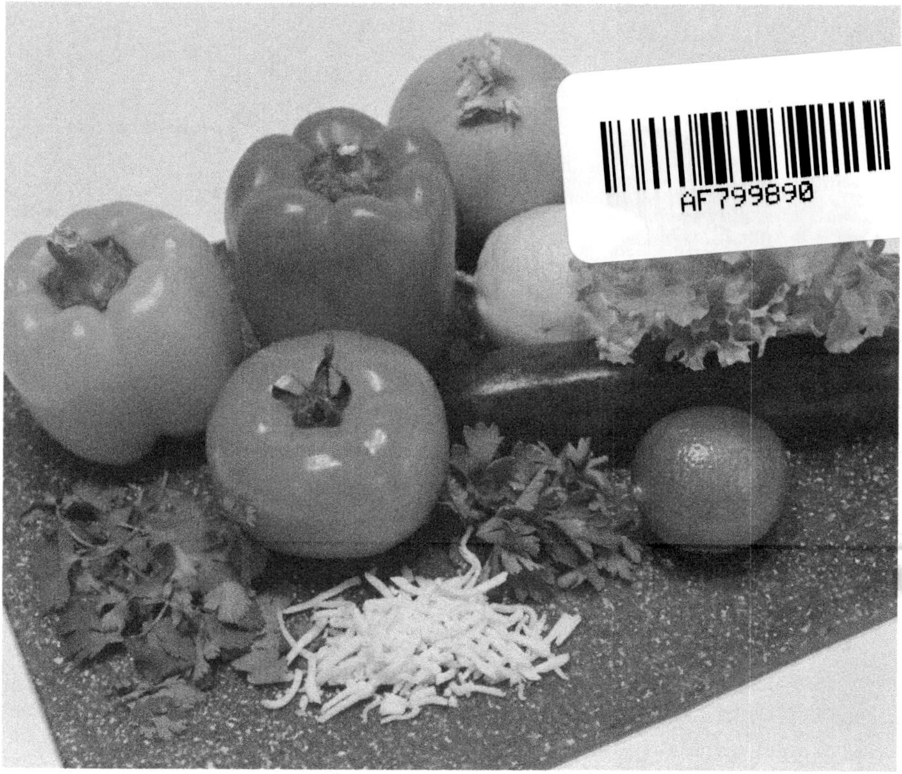

just the recipes

by the krazy keto cooks

Maudsley Publishing

Library of Congress Control Number: 2019911869
krazy keto cookbook by the krazy keto cooks
published by Maudsley Publishing, Woodbridge, VA
first edition August, 2019
https://twitter.com/keto4foodies
https://www.instagram.com/krazyketocookbook/

Cover by DAC Clark
ISBN: 978-1-7333971-0-0 (paperback)
ISBN: 978-1-7333971-1-7 (ebook)

Publisher's Note

All notes and information in this book are believed to be accurate at time of this writing. However, the author or publisher cannot accept any legal responsibility or liability for any errors or omissions that may have been made or any loss, harm or injuries that comes from following instructions or advice in this book.

to our silent partner, a fabulous taste-tester, supporter of krazy cooks, the keto diet and all-round devoted friend --and to all our family and friends, who sat and listened to us rave about our recipes.

table of contents

introduction – just the recipes

krazy keto cooks (who will be henceforth referred to as k^2c) are just about the recipes. k^2c have achieved 50 percent of our weight loss goals in just five months following the recipes in this book. watch for possible k^2c's before-and-after pictures in *krazy keto cookbook - part II.* for your convenience, we have added a note section to each recipe to allow for customizable cooking.

please read the helpful notes within the recipes for best textures and cooking hints.

on weekends, k^2c make many of these recipes to be frozen for weekly dinners, using fresh vegetables and salads to complement each meal.

the preparation times shown for the recipes are accurate once you have made the recipe a few times. k2c also use some great prepping tools, such as a veggie spiralizer and the saladshooter, to decrease the time spent preparing vegetables. we highly recommend the saladshooter for conveniently grating cheese and dicing vegetables for many of our dishes.

cooking note: parchment paper is key to success with baking items.

casserole note: baking powder allows thickening of casseroles that limits the carbohydrates in these recipes.

full disclosure: the bread section is for maintaining weight levels, not for losing further fat/weight. stick to the non-bread sections to stay on the keto diet.

thank you for purchasing our book. now for just the recipes.

visit us on twitter and instagram for the latest cooking with the k2c:

https://twitter.com/keto4foodies

https://www.instagram.com/krazyketocookbook/

luscious loaf

prep time
10 mins

cook time
35 - 40 mins

serves
48 slices

total carbs
58

things you need

6 large
eggs (beaten)

3 cups
milk at room temperature

1 stick
melted butter

3 cups
almond flour

1 1/4 cups
vital wheat gluten

6 tablespoons
spelt flour

1 teaspoon
honey

1 teaspoon
salt

1 tablespoon
truvia or stevia

2 teaspoon
yeast

2 tablespoons
baking powder

cooking instructions

1 heat oven to **375 degrees**. beat eggs. add milk and melted butter in a large mixing bowl.

2 then mix almond flour, wheat gluten, spelt flour, honey, salt, truvia, yeast and baking powder into the mixing bowl with liquid.

3 use parchment paper to line 3 medium-size bread pans. add equal amounts of batter to each pan.

4 bake in the oven for 35 – 40 minutes. remove bread from pans and place on a cooling rack. allow the bread to cool before slicing.

helpful notes

additional suggestions: for sweeter bread, add additional honey or truvia.

your notes

savory stixs

prep time
20 mins

cook time
9 mins

serves
4 to 6

total carbs
65

things you need

2 large
eggs

1/2 package
cream cheese

2 tablespoons
italian seasoning

2 teaspoons
baking powder

4 cups
shredded mozzarella

2 cups
almond flour

cooking instructions

1 in large bowl, mix eggs, cream cheese, italian seasoning, salt, pepper and baking powder.

2 in glass microwavable bowl add 4 cups mozzarella cheese and melt for 3 to 4 minutes. if not completely melted, stir and then heat another 30 seconds.

3 mix mozzarella with egg and cream cheese mixture.

4 slowly add almond flour to finish the dough mixture. once completely mixed, roll out 4-inch sticks about 1/4 of an inch in diameter.

5 place parchment paper onto a cookie sheet, then place dough sticks about 1/4-inch apart and bake in the oven 5-9 minutes at **375 degrees**. depending on your taste, breadsticks can be lightly toasted or well done. repeat to cook all dough.

helpful notes

to roll dough smoothly, use a sheet of plastic wrap between the rolling pin and the dough.

your notes

tortilla chips

prep time
20 mins

cook time
9 mins

serves
4 to 6

total carbs
75

things you need

3 cups
shredded mozzarella

1/3 package
cream cheese

2 1/2 cups
almond flour

2 large
brown eggs

2 teaspoons
baking powder

1 teaspoon
pepper

1/2 teaspoon
salt

cooking instructions

1 place mozzarella cheese in a microwavable glass bowl for 3 minutes.
2 once the cheese is well melted, mix the cream cheese into the mozzarella.
3 mix the rest of the ingredients into cheese and separate dough into 5 or 6 equal parts.
4 place one piece of dough on a working area and place plastic wrap on top, then use a rolling pin to roll the dough thinly. take a plastic knife and cut into thin triangle shapes. repeat for the remaining pieces of dough.
5 place parchment paper on a cookie sheet, then place triangle pieces ¼ inch apart and bake in the oven 5-9 minutes at **375 degrees.** depending on specific taste, chips can be lightly toasted or well done. repeat to cook all dough.

helpful notes

cumin and cayenne pepper can be added to the dough for spicier chips.

your notes

perfect pitas

prep time
20 mins

cook time
10 mins

serves
6 to 8

total carbs
75

things you need

2 large
eggs

1/2 package
cream cheese

1/2 teaspoon
salt

2 teaspoons
pepper

2 teaspoons
baking powder

1 cup
puréed spinach

4 cups
shredded mozzarella

2 cups
almond flour

cooking instructions

1 in large bowl, mix eggs, cream cheese, salt, pepper and baking powder. clean spinach, and purée in a blender. add purée to egg mixture.

2 in glass microwavable bowl, add mozzarella cheese and melt for 3 to 4 minutes. if not completely melted, then stir and heat another 30 seconds.

3 mix melted mozzarella with spinach mixture.

4 slowly add almond flour to finish the dough mixture. once completely mixed, roll out dough to 1/2-inch thickness. use a plastic knife or circle cookie cutter and cut dough into even circles.

5 place parchment paper on a cookie sheet, then place pita pieces close to each other and bake in the oven 5-9 minutes at **375 degrees**. depending on specific taste, chips can be lightly toasted or well done repeat to cook all dough.

helpful notes

to roll dough smoothly, use a sheet of plastic wrap between the rolling pin and dough. optional: add garlic and/or rosemary to make different-tasting pitas, or leave out spinach for plain pitas.

your notes

choice crackers

prep time
20 mins

cook time
9 mins

serves
6 to 8

total carbs
65

things you need

6 tablespoons
cream cheese

2 tablespoons
finely crushed rosemary

5 cloves
minced garlic

1 /4 teaspoon
salt

1/2 teaspoon
black pepper

2 teaspoons
baking powder

4 cups
shredded mozzarella

2 cups
almond flour

cooking instructions

1 these instructions are very similar to perfect pita recipe; however, these chips should be rolled thinner to make wispy crackers and does have different flavor. in a large bowl, slowly add and mix the cream cheese, rosemary seasoning, garlic, salt, pepper and baking powder.

2 in glass microwavable bowl, add mozzarella cheese and melt for 3-4 minutes. if not completely melted, stir and heat another 30 seconds.

3 mix mozzarella with cream cheese mixture.

4 slowly add almond flour to finish the dough mixture. once completely mixed, roll the dough to 1/2-inch thickness on a nonstick sheet pan.

5 cut dough into 2-inch squares. bake at **375 degrees** for 5-9 minutes to lightly brown crackers.

helpful notes

to roll dough smoothly, use a sheet of plastic wrap between the rolling pin and dough. use crackers with cheese or for small sandwiches.

your notes

phat egg sandwich

prep time
20 mins

cook time
10 mins

serves
2

total carbs
12

things you need

4 large
eggs

1 dash
sea salt to taste

1 dash
black pepper

1/2 pound
bacon strips

toppings

1/2 medium
sliced red onion

1 cup
sliced avocado

1 large
sliced vine ripe tomato

4 slices
american white cheese

cooking instructions

1 cook bacon strips and set aside.

2 slice red onions, avocado, and tomatoes and set aside.

3 in four porcelain ramekins, crack an egg in each and add desired salt and pepper. bake for 10 minutes in the oven at **375 degrees**, until completely cooked. remove eggs from oven.

4 on one of the cooked eggs, place a slice of cheese, bacon, avocado, onions and tomatoes, then add another egg on top to complete the sandwich. repeat for the second sandwich.

helpful notes

if you do not have ramekins, eggs can be cooked in a very small frying pan. additional toppings include jalapenos, chives and salsa.

your notes

breakfast

buttery blueberry delite

prep time
10 mins

cook time
25 mins

serves
3 to 4

total carbs
58

things you need

2 cups
almond flour

3 tablespoons
cream cheese

2 large
eggs

1 tablespoon
vanilla

5 tablespoons
truvia or stevia

2 teaspoons
baking powder

1/2 teaspoon
sea salt

2 tablespoons
whole cream

1/2 cup
melted butter

2 teaspoons (optional)
gluten

3/4 cup
fresh blueberries

cooking instructions

1 preheat oven to **350 degrees**. line muffin pan with muffin cups.

2 then in a large mixing bowl add dry ingredients. then add wet ingredients. make sure batter does not have cream cheese chunks. when the batter is smooth, slowly add rest of ingredients, lastly add blueberries.

3 fill muffin cups 2/3 full (6-8 servings) and bake for 25 minutes or until browned.

4 serve with additional butter.

helpful notes

additional suggestions: gluten can be removed from the recipe or add an additional 1-2 teaspoons for less crumbly muffins. forks are highly recommended for this recipe.

your notes

avocado soufflé

prep time
10 mins

cook time
~10 mins

serves
2

total carbs
37

things you need

4 large
cage-free eggs

2 large
avocados

1/2 medium
red onion

2 medium
vine ripe tomatoes

toppings

1/2 cup
grated cheddar cheese

1/2 cup
grated cheddar cheese

2 large
jalapenos

1/2 teaspoon
salsa

1/2 cup
sour cream

cooking instructions

1 dice red onion, tomato and grated cheese. slice jalapenos in half lengthwise, then slice halves into eight thin slices.

2 cut avocados in half and take out the pit.

3 place avocados in a baking dish, cut side up, then crack and place 1 egg into each half of avocado. bake avocados and eggs for ~10 minutes (depending on your desired egg type) at **400 degrees**.

4 when eggs are cooked, place the avocados on a plate and add jalapenos, red onions, tomatoes, cheddar cheese, salsa and sour cream on top.

helpful notes

optional: bacon and green onions can be substituted for topping ingredients.

your notes

fluffy pancakes

prep time
5 mins

cook time
15 mins

serves
3 to 4

total carbs
60

things you need

2 cups
almond flour

1/2 tablespoon
truvia or stevia

2 teaspoons
baking powder

2 large
eggs

1 tablespoon
vanilla

1/3 package
softened cream cheese

1 cup
water (to desired pancake thickness)

toppings

2 tablespoons
sugar-free syrup

1/2 stick
Butter

cooking instructions

1 mix flour, truvia and baking powder. in a large bowl, mix together eggs, vanilla and cream cheese, ensuring there are no lumps.

2 add flour to the wet ingredients. when the batter is smooth, slowly add water (may need more or less water depending on desired consistency).

3 best to grill in a nonstick pan on **medium heat**.

4 use sugar-free syrup and regular butter for toppings. Dollar size pancakes are preferred.

helpful notes

add more vanilla or cinnamon to the batter to taste. pancakes freeze for an on-the-run breakfast.

your notes

sausage egg soufflé

prep time
10 mins

cook time
35 mins

serves
6 to 8

total carbs
52

things you need

1 pound
cooked breakfast sausage
(spicy optional)

12 large
brown eggs

1/2 cup
cheddar cheese

1/2 cup
mozzarella cheese

1/4 cup
almond flour

1 medium
yellow onion, diced

toppings

1 teaspoon
black pepper

1 cup
chopped spinach

1 chopped
ripe vine tomato

1/2 cup
finely chopped chives

2 large
avocados

1/2 cup
sour cream

cooking instructions

1 chop the sausage into 1/2-inch pieces and place in casserole dish.

2 in a separate bowl, beat the eggs, then add mozzarella cheese, almond flour, onion, pepper and spinach, and stir until mixture is smooth. pour mixture over sausage. sprinkle cheddar cheese on top of casserole.

3 place casserole dish in the oven for 35 mins at **375 degrees**.

4 chop tomato, chives and avocados for toppings while casserole cooks.

5 serve tomatoes, chives, avocados, and sour cream on top of each portion.

helpful notes

bacon can be substituted for sausage. for a dryer soufflé, drain half of the fat from sausage before mixing in casserole.

your notes

baked tilapia

prep time
20 mins

cook time
45 mins

serves
6 to 8

total carbs
6

things you need

6-8 fillets
tilapia fish

7-9 cloves
minced garlic

1 medium
diced yellow onion

4-6 tablespoons
butter

2 tablespoons
italian dressing

2 tablespoons
italian seasoning

1/2 teaspoon
black pepper

2 teaspoons
baking powder

2 tablespoons
almond flour

6-8 tablespoons
parmesan cheese

cooking instructions

1 place tilapia fillets in a nonstick baking dish.

2 mix garlic, onion and butter and microwave for 30-40 seconds.

3 combine the butter mixture with the italian dressing, italian seasoning, pepper, baking powder and almond flour and drizzle over tilapia fillets. sprinkle parmesan cheese on top of fillets.

4 bake at **375 degrees** for 35-45 minutes - cooked medium to well done.

5 serve with salad or green beans.

helpful notes

be certain to bake thoroughly to prevent undercooking. cooking time varies depending on the type of oven used. also may be served with asparagus.

your notes

chicken tenders

prep time
20 mins

cook time
15 mins

serves
4 to 6

total carbs
64

things you need

1/2 cup
mayonnaise

1 tablespoon
salt and pepper to taste

8 cloves
minced garlic

1 large
diced yellow onion

1 1/2 cups
shredded parmesan cheese

4 large
chicken breasts, cut in 4-inch

4 cups
chopped organic cauliflower

1/2 stick
butter

2 cups
olive oil

2 cups
almond flour

cooking instructions

1 mix mayonnaise, salt and pepper, 4 cloves garlic, onion, 1 cup parmesan cheese and cut chicken in a gallon-size ziplock bag. set aside.

2 steam cauliflower until desired tenderness. spread chunks of butter evenly over cauliflower in baking pan and top remaining garlic and cheese. place in the oven to bake 10-15 minutes at **375 degrees**.

3 in a nonstick skillet, add oil and heat on medium for 3-5 minutes. place almond flour in a shallow dish and slowly add chicken marinade, coat the chicken pieces in the flour, and then pan-fry chicken tenders until golden brown.

helpful notes

serve roasted cauliflower and chicken with ranch dressing and green leaf lettuce if desired.

your notes

american

stuffed peppers/meatloaf

prep time
20 mins

cook time
45 mins

serves
6 to 8

total carbs
88

things you need

7 cloves
minced garlic

1 large
white onion, diced

1/2 cup
almond flour

4 large
brown eggs

1 teaspoon
pepper

1 teaspoon
salt (to taste)

3 tablespoons
italian seasoning

3 pounds
ground beef (85%)

8 large
green peppers or colored peppers

16 ounces
mozzarella cheese

sides

1 can
organic tomato sauce

3 cans or 1 pound fresh
green beans or asparagus

cooking instructions

1 slowly sauté garlic and onion lightly for 5 minutes in a saucepan. then in large bowl, mix almond flour, eggs, salt, pepper, italian seasoning, ground beef and sautéed vegetables.

2 cut peppers in half, remove seeds and wash. in a glass baking dish place peppers and fill with meat mixture. pour tomato sauce over peppers and add mozzarella cheese on top.

3 bake peppers for 45 minutes at **375 degrees**.

4 10 minutes before peppers are finished cooking, sauté or steam green beans or asparagus.

helpful notes

if peppers are not desired, create meatloaf instead, cooking at **375 degrees** for 60 minutes.

your notes

mesquite burgers

prep time
15 mins

cook time
12 mins

serves
6 to 8

total carbs
34

things you need

1 medium
yellow onion, diced

3 pounds
ground beef (85%)

2 tablespoons
mesquite seasoning

2 teaspoons
salt

2 teaspoons
pepper

toppings

1 head
green lettuce or bok choy (cleaned and uncut)

1 small
red onion, sliced thinly

2 small
tomatoes, sliced thinly

2 large
sliced avocados

8 slices
pepper jack cheese

cooking instructions

1 dice yellow onions, slice red onions thinly, slice tomatoes thinly and peel/slice avocados into wedges. set all aside in the refrigerator.

2 clean bok choy/lettuce leaves well and set aside to dry.

3 gently mix ground beef (do not knead excessively), diced yellow onions and all seasonings in a large mixing bowl. then make round patties approximately 1 to 1 1/2 inches thick. best if **grilled** on outside grill 6-7 minutes on each side.

4 when burgers are done, place patties between lettuce/bok choy leaves and top with desired fresh vegetables and pepper jack cheese.

helpful notes

low-carb wraps may be used instead of lettuce wraps. optional: add pickles, jalapenos, sautéed mushrooms, blue cheese or bacon to the burger.

your notes

tuna zoodles

prep time
20 mins

cook time
10 mins

serves
6 to 8

total carbs
124

things you need

2 cans
solid white tuna in water

1/3 cup
mayonnaise

1 32-ounce can
mushroom soup

1 tablespoon
mild curry

1/2 teaspoon
pepper

1 tablespoon
cornstarch

2 cups
chopped celery

1 medium
white onion, chopped

3 pounds
zucchini noodles

1 12-ounce can
drained green peas (do not use frozen)

3 cups
broccoli

1 pound
grated cheddar cheese

cooking instructions

1 slowly add drained tuna, mayonnaise, mushroom soup, curry and pepper to a pot and slowly heat. mix in cornstarch. the sauce should be creamy and thick, not thin.

2 dice celery and onions into ½-inches. use a zoodle maker on the thickest setting to cut the zucchini. once tuna sauce is hot and has desired taste, add onion, celery, peas and broccoli.

3 cook sauce 5 minutes, then add tuna sauce to a glass baking dish. layer zoodles over the top. cover zoodles with cheese, bake 10 minutes at **425 degrees**.

helpful notes

optional: add 1/2 a cup of parmesan and romano cheese with the cheddar cheese before baking. note, for less of a crunchy texture, sauté the onions and celery to desired softness. curry can be removed for a more traditional american taste. for less crunchy vegetables, cook for extra 10-15 minutes.

reference: zoodle maker is a vegetable spiralizer; see link for more details: **https://en.wikipedia.org/wiki/spiral_vegetable_slicer**

your notes

italian

chicken parmesan

prep time
20 mins

cook time
30 mins

serves
4 to 6

total carbs
71

things you need

1/2 stick
butter

10 cloves
minced garlic

1 medium
yellow onion

1 teaspoon
black pepper

2 pounds
chicken breast

2 cups
zucchini noodles

2 cups
spaghetti sauce, preferred organic

1/2 cup
grated parmesan cheese

4 ounces
shredded mozzarella cheese

side

2 cups
broccoli

cooking instructions

1 in a large skillet on **low heat**, add butter, garlic, onion and pepper. cook on low heat for 10 minutes.

2 cut chicken into thinly sliced 2-inch long pieces.

3 add chicken to the skillet over medium heat. grill chicken 15 minutes until medium brown.

4 place cooked chicken in bottom of glass baking dish, place zoodles on top of chicken. add preferred spaghetti sauce, then parmesan and mozzarella cheese.

5 bake dish for 15 minutes at **400 degrees**.

6 steam broccoli while the dish is cooking.

helpful notes

if crunch is preferred on vegetables, then steam broccoli for no more than 7-9 minutes. if zucchini is preferred crunchy, then place zoodles and cheeses on top of the dish after 5 minutes of cooking chicken in oven first.

your notes

italian

chicken alfredo

prep time
20 mins

cook time
25 mins

serves
4 to 6

total carbs
34

things you need

1/2 stick
butter

10 cloves
minced garlic

1 medium
yellow onion, chopped

1 teaspoon
black pepper

2 pounds
chicken breast

2 cups
zucchini noodles

2 cups
broccoli

8 ounces
cream cheese

1 cup
grated parmesan cheese

1 to 2 cups
water

1 cup
shredded mozzarella cheese

cooking instructions

1 in a large skillet on **low heat**, add butter, garlic, onion and pepper. cook on low heat for 10 minutes.

2 cut chicken into thin slices, 1 to 2 inches long. add chicken to the skillet over medium heat. cook chicken 15 minutes. stir occasionally.

3 while the chicken is cooking, spiralize 2 cups of zucchini and cut up 2 cups of broccoli.

4 slowly add cream cheese and parmesan cheese with 1 cup of water, then slowly add mozzarella. stir continuously.

5 once sauce thins somewhat, add zoodles and broccoli to skillet cover for 5 minutes to steam.

helpful notes

the cream sauce can be made in a separate saucepan and added to the chicken after it is cooked. for more tender broccoli, add it to the skillet while the chicken is cooking.

your notes

veggie pizza

prep time
20 mins

cook time
10 mins

serves
6 to 8

total carbs
125

things you need

7 cloves
minced garlic

1 large
yellow onion

2 large
green peppers

4 tablespoons
italian seasoning

2 large
brown eggs

6 tablespoons
cream cheese

2 teaspoons
baking powder

4 cups
shredded mozzarella

2 cups
almond flour

toppings

4 cups
organic spaghetti sauce

3 cups
shredded mozzarella

cooking instructions

1 slowly sauté garlic, onion, green peppers and 2 tablespoons of italian seasoning. then in large bowl, mix eggs, cream cheese, 2 tablespoons of italian seasoning and baking powder.

2 in glass microwavable bowl, add 4 cups mozzarella cheese and melt for 3 minutes. stir and, if not completely melted, heat another 30 seconds.

3 mix mozzarella with the egg and cream cheese mixture.

4 slowly add almond flour to finish the dough mixture. once completely mixed, place parchment paper on a nonstick sheet pan, and roll out dough to 4-inch-wide pizzas, to desired thickness.

5 spread 4 cups of spaghetti sauce over the pizza and sprinkle remaining mozzarella cheese on top. bake 8 to 10 minutes to desired crispness at **425 degrees**.

helpful notes

to roll dough smoothly, use a sheet of plastic wrap between the rolling pin and dough. add sautéed mushrooms or other toppings as desired. when making dough, be sure to make pizzas no larger than 4 inches so the crust is crispy. when looking for spaghetti sauces, look for low-sugar, low-carb versions.

your notes

italian

shrimp scampi

prep time
25 mins

cook time
5-7 mins

serves
6 to 8

total carbs
22

things you need

1 pound
shrimp

1 medium
lemon

1/2 stick
butter

6 cloves
minced garlic

1 teaspoon
crushed red peppers

2 tablespoons
italian seasoning

toppings

1 medium
sliced onion

1/2 cup
chopped parsley

1/2 cup
grated parmesan cheese

2 cups
zucchini noodles

cooking instructions

1 to grill, make an aluminum foil tray. put shrimp on skewers. dash crushed red peppers on top. squeeze both halves of fresh lemon over shrimp.

2 dice up butter and garlic and sprinkle over shrimp skewers.

3 put aluminum foil tray on the grill, making sure not to poke holes in the tray. once the butter begins to sizzle and shrimp is cooked, the bottom side will have a white line about halfway up.

4 flip the shrimp and cook the other side. this should only take 5-7 minutes. once done, remove skewers from tray. carefully drain butter into a small dish and use for dipping if desired.

5 add the desired level of veggies, such as grilled zucchini, yellow squash and peppers. if using zucchini noodles, parsley or sliced onions, sauté in skillet for 2-3 minutes. top with grated parmesan cheese.

helpful notes

directions for italian stir-fry: in a frying pan, melt butter with garlic, and cook until sizzling. while butter is melting, squeeze both halves of lemon over shrimp, then add to sizzling butter. sprinkle with a couple of dashes of crushed red pepper. stir shrimp to make sure they are not overcooked.

the shrimp should be done in 5-7 minutes. remove shrimp with a slotted spoon, drain butter sauce into a small dish, use for dipping if desired. can also be served with cocktail sauce.

your notes

____

____

____

____

italian sausage spaghetti

prep time
15 mins

cook time
35 mins

serves
6 to 8

total carbs
56

things you need

1 tablespoon

butter

8 cloves

minced garlic

1/2 medium

yellow onion

1 1/2 teaspoons

black pepper

1 package

italian sausage (hot/spicy)

2 tablespoons

italian seasoning

2 tablespoons

oregano

2 8oz cans

of hunt's tomato sauce

2 tablespoons

hunt's tomato paste

1-2 cups

filtered water

2 cups

zucchini noodles

1 tablespoon

olive oil

optional

salt

to taste after
adding sausage

cooking instructions

1 in a large skillet on **medium-low heat**, add butter garlic, onion and 1 teaspoon of pepper. reduce heat and cook on low for 5 minutes.

2 peel skin from sausages and cut them into 1-inch chunks.

3 add sausage and dry seasonings to separate skillet; cook on medium heat for 15 minutes.

4 add hunt's sauce and paste with water to a saucepan. drain grease from skillet, then add the sausage to spaghetti sauce, add salt to taste, and cook for 30 minutes on **medium heat**.

5 once the sauce is cooked, add zoodles to a skillet with olive oil and 1/2 teaspoon pepper and cover for 2-3 minutes to steam.

helpful notes

for a sweeter sauce, add 1 teaspoon of stevia or truvia. ensure that sausage is thoroughly cooked in a skillet prior to adding to the saucepan. for al dente noodles, steam 1 minute.

your notes

beef tostadas

prep time
10 mins

cook time
30 mins

serves
3 to 4

total carbs
38

special note: use the perfect pita recipe for the tostadas. they should be prepped beforehand, either fresh or frozen. see the bread section for perfect pita recipe.

things you need

1 pound

85% organic ground beef

1 package

favorite taco seasoning

1-2 cups

filtered water

2 medium

avocados

1/2 medium

diced red onion

1 cup

chopped cilantro

toppings

1 medium

diced yellow onion

4 cloves

minced garlic

1 cup

favorite salsa

2 cups

organic roma tomatoes

1/4 cup

diced jalapenos

cooking instructions

1 in a large skillet on **medium-low heat**, add garlic, yellow onion, and ground beef. cook on low heat for 15 minutes. while cooking, with a fork break up ground beef to mix in onion and garlic to make ground beef smaller. add taco seasoning and water. cook another 15 minutes until well done.

2 while the meat is cooking, dice red onions, tomatoes, cilantro.and jalapenos. peel and slice avocados.

3 add cooked meat to warm keto tostadas/pita; add salsa and desired toppings.

helpful notes

for additional toppings, add cheddar cheese and/or sour cream on top. keto tostadas that are frozen should be reheated at **400 degrees** for 5-7 minutes.

your notes

mexican

chicken enchiladas

prep time
15 mins

cook time
35 mins

serves
6 to 8

total carbs
100

things you need

2 pounds

chicken

1 tablespoon

cumin

10-ounce can

organic enchilada sauce

1 medium

yellow onion

6 cloves

minced garlic

2 large

zucchini

toppings

1 pound

grated sharp cheddar cheese

1 bunch

diced green onions

1 cup

sour cream

4 cups

lettuce

1 cup

cilantro

3-4 large

avocados

cooking instructions

1 in a large skillet on medium-low heat, add chicken, cumin, enchilada sauce, onions and garlic. cook for 35 minutes, stirring occasionally.

2 while the chicken is cooking, peel zucchini, cut it in half and then slice thinly. set oven to **400 degrees**. salt zucchini slices and place on parchment paper on a cookie sheet and bake for 15-20 minutes to dry zucchini. alternatively, baking in air fry will take less time.

3 in a glass baking dish, lay zucchini flat to cover the bottom of the dish, add chicken and half of the enchilada sauce, and layer any remaining zucchini on top. add rest of sauce, cheese and diced green onions.

4 put glass dish in the oven and bake for 10 minutes. for crispier cheese topping, cook up to 20 minutes.

5 serve topped with sour cream, lettuce, diced cilantro and avocado slices.

helpful notes

for spicier taste, add diced habanero peppers on top. chicken can also be cooked longer or in a crockpot for shredded chicken texture.

your notes

mexican

chicken tortilla soup

prep time
15 mins

cook time
45 mins

serves
6 to 8

total carbs
121

things you need

2 pounds

chicken breast

1 can

rotel tomato sauce

2-3 cups

filtered water

1 large

jalapeno pepper

1 ½ teaspoons

black pepper

2 tablespoons

cumin

2 cubes

chicken broth broth

1 large

yellow onion

8 cloves

minced garlic

salt

to taste after cooking 20 minutes

1 tablespoon

virgin olive oil

2 tablespoons

chili powder

1 cup

pinto beans

toppings

diced **cilantro**

shredded **cheddar/pepper jack**

chunks of **avocado**

chopped **red onions**

cooking instructions

1 in a large pot on **medium heat**, add all ingredients to the pot, except pinto beans and noted toppings.

2 in smaller pot, cook pinto beans in water until tender. when tender, drain beans, then add beans to the pot of soup. bring to a boil, then reduce to low and cook for 45 minutes.

3 while the soup is cooking, prepare toppings.

4 after 20-30 minutes, test the taste of the soup; add salt if desired.

5 at around 35 minutes, start to pull apart chicken so it is either shredded or in smaller pieces. serve the soup with toppings.

helpful notes

for spicier taste, add diced habanero peppers on top.

your notes

mexican

cilantro beef chili

prep time
15-30 mins

cook time
1 hour

serves
8 to 10

total carbs
121

things you need

1 cup

pinto beans

1/4 cup

virgin olive oil

2 1/2 to 3 pounds

1-inch-by-1-inch sliced shoulder roast

1 large

chopped yellow onion

8 cloves

minced garlic

2 large

chopped green/red peppers

2 or 3 fresh

chopped chili pods (yellow)

3 tablespoons

chili powder

2 teaspoons

oregano

1 teaspoon

cayenne pepper

2 teaspoons

black pepper

1 large

bay leaf

3 tablespoons

cornstarch

6-8 cups

filtered water

1 cube

beef bouillon

4 teaspoons

truvia

salt

to taste

toppings

diced **cilantro**

chopped **red onion**

sliced **avocados**

shredded **sharp cheddar**

cooking instructions

1 soak beans overnight or cook in salted water, following directions on the package, for approximately 45 minutes or until tender.

2 heat olive oil in a large heavy skillet or dutch oven. add meat, frequently stirring. add the chopped onion, garlic, bell pepper and yellow chili. then, after combining all of the dry spices in a bowl and mixing them thoroughly, add the dry spices and the bay leaf to the pot. stir well and sauté for about 5 minutes. stir in the almond flour, blending well. add water and beef bouillon and bring to a boil. **reduce heat and simmer about 40 minutes**.

3 stir in the truvia and salt to taste. drain the beans and add to the skillet. simmer about 10 minutes longer, then serve.

4 serve in a bowl with toppings as desired.

helpful notes

depending on the type of chili peppers used, beef chili may be very spicy. use mild jalapenos or none for less spicy chili.

your notes

mexican chicken salad

prep time
15 mins

cook time
35 mins

serves
6 to 8

total carbs
68

things you need

1 tablespoon

fresh diced jalapeno

10 cloves

minced garlic

1 large

diced yellow onion

2 pounds

organic chicken

2 tablespoons

cumin

2 tablespoons

chili powder

1 cup

water

1 can

rotel tomato sauce

1 cube

chicken bouillon

salt

to taste

toppings

chopped **lettuce**

sliced **avocados**

sour cream

salsa

diced **tomatoes**

diced **red onions**

shredded **cheddar cheese**

cooking instructions

1 in a large pot on **medium-low heat**, add jalapenos, diced garlic, diced onion, chicken, cumin, chili powder, water, rotel tomato sauce and chicken bouillon. increase heat to medium and cook for 35 minutes.
2 dice tomatoes and red onions. shred cheese. chop lettuce and slice avocados. set all aside.
3 pull chicken apart as it is cooking. add salt to taste. ideally, most of the water should cook off.
4 once the chicken is completely cooked, add chicken to a bowl of salad with sliced avocados.
5 add additional toppings as desired.

helpful notes

extra chicken can be frozen for lunches or dinners.

your notes

beef kebobs

prep time
20 mins

cook time
15 mins

serves
6 to 8

total carbs
25

things you need

3 large

yellow onions

3 pounds

ground beef (85%)

2 tablespoons

salt

1 tablespoon

black pepper

1 tablespoon

baking soda

5-7 medium

tomatoes

yogurt

2 cups

yogurt (whole milk plain)

1 cup

cubed cucumbers

1/2 teaspoon

salt to taste

3 cloves

diced garlic

cooking instructions

1 use a hand grater to grate peeled onions into a large bowl. add ground beef, salt, pepper and baking soda. mix well. set aside.

2 dice cucumbers and garlic. in a glass bowl, add yogurt, garlic, cucumbers and salt. place in the refrigerator.

3 make 4-inch-long kebobs and cook on the grill or frying pan **medium heat** for 15 minutes adding sliced tomatoes after 10 minutes.

4 serve kebobs with grilled tomatoes and yogurt.

helpful notes

optional: beef, tomatoes and yogurt can be added to low-carb pitas. recommend salad shirazi to complement.

your notes

cornish hen

prep time
20 mins

cook time
20 mins

serves
6 to 8

total carbs
96

things you need

2 small

cornish hens

1 large

white onion

1 teaspoon

granulated saffron

1 medium

lemon

1/2 cup

olive oil

1/2 teaspoon each

salt and pepper to taste

2 large

tomatoes, halved

sides

4 cups

fresh green beans

1/2 teaspoon

salt and pepper to taste

yogurt dip:

2 cups

yogurt (whole milk greek plain)

1 cup

cubed cucumbers

3 pieces

minced garlic

1/2 teaspoon

salt and pepper to taste

cooking instructions

1 cut cornish hen in 4-6 pieces, grate onion into a bowl and add meat, saffron, lemon, olive oil and salt/pepper to taste. mix and leave the meat to marinate overnight in the refrigerator.

2 in a glass bowl, bake or grill cornish hen with halved tomatoes for 20 minutes at **400 degrees**. while hens are cooking, sauté green beans on low in olive oil with salt and pepper to taste.

3 chop cucumbers and garlic, and mix them with yogurt. season with salt and pepper to taste.

4 serve hens with green beans and yogurt on the side.

helpful notes

for yogurt, add fresh diced mint or dill for additional flavor. optional: add shirazi salad with the meal. cornish hen may be switched with chicken

optional: use 3-to-4-pound roasting chicken.

your notes

persian

eggplant lettuce wraps

prep time
20 mins

cook time
10 mins

serves
6 to 8

total carbs
96

things you need

2 large

eggplants

1 tablespoon

turmeric

2 large

tomatoes

1 large

white onion

1 large

yellow onion

1/2 teaspoon each

salt and pepper to taste

10 cloves

minced garlic

8 - 12 tablespoons

olive oil

1 head

bok choy or lettuce

8 spears

chilled dill pickles

1/2 bunch

parsley

1 pound

cubed feta cheese

cooking instructions

1 peel skin from eggplant and slice into 1/2-inch round slices. to dry eggplant, place a paper towel on a plate, then place a layer of eggplant on the paper towel; lightly salt and cover with a paper towel then add another layer of eggplant. repeat until all eggplant is lightly salted and covered. dry out overnight if possible, in a large ziplock bag or sealed container.

2 slice tomatoes into wedges. cut white onion and yellow onion in half then thinly slice.

3 in nonstick pan, slowly sauté yellow onion, garlic and eggplant in olive oil. eggplant should be thoroughly fried. add sliced tomatoes and turmeric to the pan. cook an additional 10 minutes. once hot, serve with chilled pickles, parsley, feta cheese, sliced white onions and wrap in lettuce leaf.

helpful notes

yogurt or shirazi salad can be added to complement.

your notes

herb quiche

prep time
20 mins

cook time
15 mins

serves
6 to 8

total carbs
89

things you need

1 full bag

spinach

1 bunch

cilantro

2 bunches

parsley

1 large

diced yellow onion

9 large

brown eggs

1/2 teaspoon

salt

1 teaspoon

black pepper

1/2 cup

olive oil

1 tablespoon

turmeric

1 container

baby tomatoes

1 jar

kosher sandwich pickles

yogurt mix

2 cups

yogurt (whole milk greek plain)

3 pieces

diced garlic

1 or 2

cubed cucumbers

1/2 teaspoon

salt to taste

cooking instructions

1 clean and soak spinach, cilantro and parsley to remove all dirt. remove leaves and dispose of branches. place vegetables on a towel to dry for 30 minutes to 1 hour or (recommended) dry them with lettuce spinner. dice all veggies well.

2 in a large bowl, mix diced onions, diced vegetables and eggs. add salt, pepper and turmeric. mix well.

3 dice cucumbers and garlic and in a glass bowl, combine yogurt, garlic, cucumbers and a pinch of salt. place in the refrigerator.

4 in a large skillet, add olive oil and cook the vegetable mixture **on low heat** for 10 minutes. while cooking, slice vegetable mixture in pie slices. flip slices over to cook for 10 additional minutes. make sure inside is well done.

5 serve herb quiche slices with fresh or grilled tomatoes and yogurt.

helpful notes

option: serve with pickles, feta cheese and fresh mint.

your notes

beef cutlets

prep time
20 mins

cook time
15 mins

serves
6 to 8

total carbs
39

things you need

3 large
yellow onions

7 large cloves
minced garlic

3 pounds
ground beef (85%)

1 teaspoon
salt to taste

1/2 tablespoon
black pepper

1 tablespoon
turmeric

2-4 large
tomatoes

1 bunch
fresh green mint and parsley

8-12 ounces
feta cheese, cubed

yogurt mix

2 cups
yogurt (whole greek plain)

1 cup
cubed cucumbers

3 cloves
minced garlic

1/2 teaspoon
salt to taste

cooking instructions

1 grate peeled onions and garlic into a large bowl. add ground beef, salt, pepper and turmeric. mix well.

2 dice cucumbers, garlic and in a glass bowl, combine yogurt, garlic, cucumbers and salt. place in the refrigerator. clean herbs and let dry.

3 make 4-inch patties and cook on the grill or frying pan for 15 minutes, adding sliced tomatoes after 10 minutes.

4 serve cutlets with grilled tomatoes, yogurt, herbs and feta cheese on top.

helpful notes

optional: cutlets can be served in a large lettuce leaf or bok choy leaf to make a wrap.

your notes

anti-pasta salad

prep time
20 mins

chill time
1 hour

serves
6 to 8

total carbs
53

things you need

3 cups

raw cauliflower

2 cups

raw broccoli

2 medium

tomatoes

1 medium

red pepper

1 medium

red onion

10 slices

salami

20 slices

pepperoni

10 slices

ham

2 cups

diced provolone or parmesan cheese

6 tablespoons

vinaigrette dressing

1 tablespoon

italian seasoning

1 tablespoon

olive oil

cooking instructions

1 on a cutting board, chop up and slice all vegetables into the ~1/4-inch pieces.

2 on cutting board, slice cold meats into 1-inch slices.

3 in large glass bowl, mix vegetables, cold meats and shredded cheese with vinaigrette dressing, italian seasoning and olive oil.

4 chill salad in the refrigerator for at least 1 hour. it can also be chilled overnight.

helpful notes

your notes

ceviche shrimp salad

prep time
20 mins

cook time
3-5 mins

serves
6 to 8

total carbs
46

things you need

1 pound

jumbo shrimp

4 medium

diced ripe vine tomatoes

1 medium

lemon

3 large

diced ripe avocados

1-2 medium

diced jalapenos

2 large

minced garlic cloves

sauce

1 large

yellow onion (to taste)

4 tablespoons

ketchup

2 tablespoons

horseradish

1/3 medium

squeezed lemon

1/2 - 1 teaspoon

salt (to taste)

1/2 - 1 teaspoon

pepper (to taste)

cooking instructions

1 bring a pot of water to a boil - cook shrimp 3-4 minutes. better to undercook shrimp than to overcook.
2 prepare other ingredients as specified.
3 chill shrimp for 35 minutes in the refrigerator.
4 mix ingredients with the chilled shrimp and serve with sauce.

helpful notes

this dish is best served chilled 2-3 hours. jalapenos are optional if there's an aversion to spicy. for party splurging, serve with tortilla chips from our bread section.

your notes

greek salad

prep time
20 mins

cook time
10 mins

serves
6 to 8

total carbs
6

things you need

4-6 large

chicken breasts

2 tablespoons

italian dressing

7 cloves

garlic

1 tablespoon

basil

1 tablespoon

dill

2 tablespoons

oregano

1 tablespoon

parsley

1 tablespoon

rosemary

1/2 tablespoon

thyme

1/2 tablespoon

black pepper

toppings

1 tablespoon

lemon pepper seasoning

1/2 tablespoon

marjoram

6 tablespoons

vinegar

1 large

chopped cucumber

1 large

red onion

1 cup

feta cheese

3 cups

shredded mozzarella

4 tablespoons

virgin olive oil

1 head

chopped lettuce

cooking instructions

1 place basil, dill, oregano, parsley, rosemary, thyme, pepper, 1/4 of italian dressing, chopped garlic and chopped onion in the skillet.

2 place chopped (1/2-inch cubes) chicken breasts into the skillet until cooked (15-20 minutes) on medium heat.

3 in a small bowl, mix lemon pepper seasoning and marjoram with virgin olive oil and vinegar.

4 serve chicken over chopped salad, chopped cucumber and cheeses.

5 serve oil and vinegar dressing mix over chicken and salad.

helpful notes

add additional virgin olive oil and vinegar to make more dressing.

your notes

shiraz salad

prep time
20 min

cook time
n/a

serves
4 to 6

total carbs
12

things you need

4 long

english hothouse cucumbers

4 large

vine ripe tomatoes

1 medium

red onion

1/4 cup

olive oil

1 large

fresh lemon

1 cup

red wine vinegar

1/2 teaspoon

salt

1/2 teaspoon

black pepper

cooking instructions

1 peel and dice cucumbers in 1/4 inch cubes.

2 finely dice red onions.

3 dice tomatoes into 1/3-inch pieces, just slightly bigger than cucumbers.

4 combine all veggies in a glass bowl, add olive oil, lemon juice, red wine vinegar, salt and pepper. mix well.

5 place salad in the refrigerator for an hour to chill.

helpful notes

optional: add dry dill to the salad for additional flavor. salad goes well with persian dishes.

your notes

sirloin napa salad

prep time
15 mins

cook time
12 mins

serves
3 to 5

total carbs
18

things you need

2 cups

worcestershire sauce

1/2 cup

olive oil

1 teaspoon

lemon juice

2 tablespoons

italian seasoning

2-4 steaks

rib eye or nyc sirloin

1 medium tightly wrapped

napa cabbage lettuce

1/2 pound

plum tomatoes

1 small

red onion

2 ounces

toppings

feta cheese

2 large

hard-boiled eggs, chopped

2-4 ounces

crumbled prosciutto (deli)

buttermilk dressing

1 tablespoon of soy sauce

1/2 teaspoon dijon mustard

3 teaspoons horseradish

2 teaspoons chives

1/2 teaspoon black pepper

1 cup buttermilk

1 cup sour cream

1/2 cup mayonnaise

cooking instructions

1 marinade includes worcestershire sauce, olive oil, lemon juice and italian seasoning.
2 slice steak into 1-inch strips and marinate for 2 hours.
3 mix together ingredients for buttermilk dressing – chill for at least 1 hour.
4 sear steak on grill for 4-6 minutes on each side.
5 cut napa cabbage into 4 wedges (rinse thoroughly), serve with drizzled dressing, tomatoes, feta cheese, egg, and prosciutto, and top with seared steak.

helpful notes

sear steak to preferred temperature. for additional spicy tastes, add additional dijon mustard and horseradish to taste.

your notes

sample menu

weekly menu planner

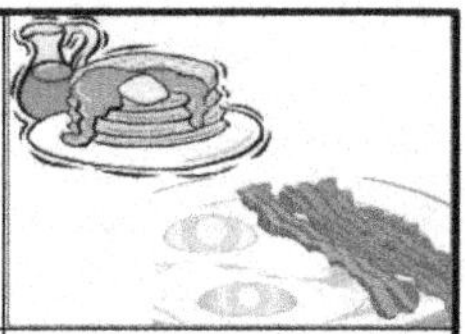

weekday	breakfast	lunch	dinner
monday	fluffy pancakes	tuna zoodles	chicken alfredo
tuesday	avocado soufflé	mesquite burgers	chicken enchiladas
wednesday	buttery blueberry delite	shrimp scampi	veggie pizza
thursday	sausage egg soufflé	chicken parmesan	sirloin napa salad
friday	phat egg sandwich	chicken tortilla soup	stuffed peppers/meatloaf
saturday	fluffy pancakes	beef kebobs	crusted baked tilapia
sunday	avocado soufflé	beef tostadas	cornish hen

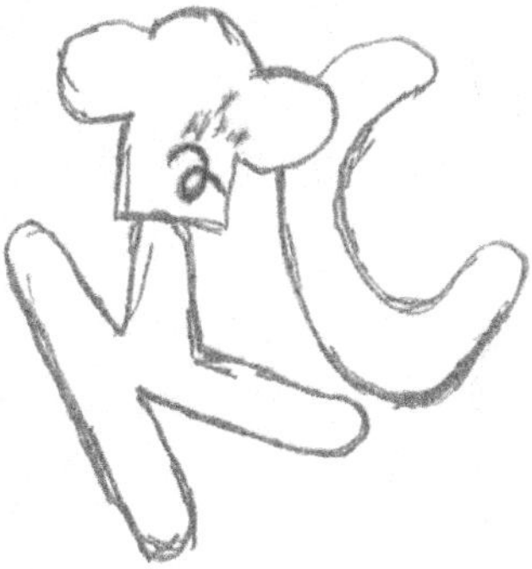

index

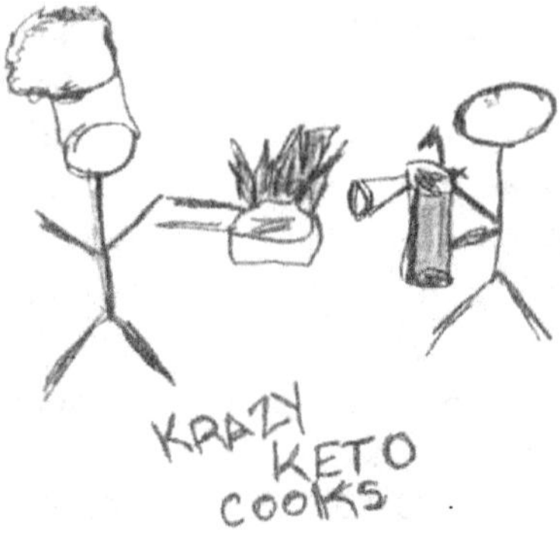
KRAZY
KETO
COOKS

Made in the USA
Monee, IL
04 November 2026

67387907R00046